Aphrodisiac's
Proven Sex Boosters For Men & Women That Work !
By Tony Xhudo M.S., H.N.
Board Certified by A. A. D. P.

Aphrodisiacs
By Tony Xhudo M.S., H.N. Board Certified by A.A.D.P.
Copyright 2012 Dawn Xhudo

Disclaimer

The information provided for you in this book is for informational purposes only and should be taken as such and is based on research by the author. This book should not be substituted as treatment or be used as such .The author and publisher of this material presented in this book are not responsible in any manner whatsoever for any harm or injury that may occur through following any information presented in this material. The information of this material is merely for educational purposes only. It is also important for the reader to consult with a health care practitioner before taking any advice contained in this book.

Dedication

I would like to dedicate this book to my wife "Dawn" for her help in all of my endeavors in my pursuit in Holistic Medicine in reaching out to those interested in Natural Health.

I love you hunny and thank you for always being there for me, even through the difficult times we shared as a couple !

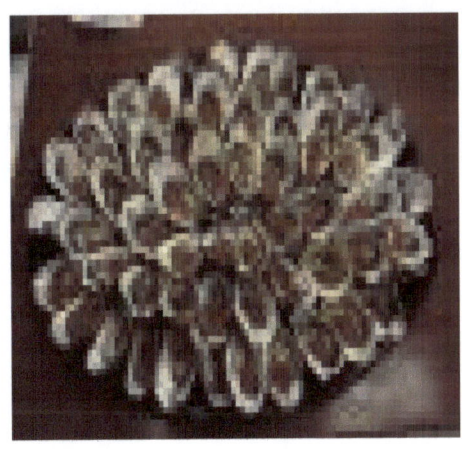

Aphrodisiacs Proven Sex Boosters

Throughout history, we have always been searching for that magic something to get ourselves and partners in the mood. For as long as humans have been having sex,they have tried everything from goat's testicles boiled in milk to silk worm extracts. As for the Food & Drug Administration,they have declared that there is no scientific proof that any over the counter aphrodisiac works to treat sexual dysfunction while knowing that their findings clash with a 5,000 year old tradition of pursuing sexual betterment through the use of foods, drugs, herbs, and magic.

Just about every culture devotes its sexual folk lore to sexual matters, and the popular issue among men and women has always been Aphrodisiacs. Whether they come from certain foods or herbs that can increase their sexual desires or libido, aphrodisiacs have always been an issue if they work or not. But believe it or not there is some truth to the matter on what does work and what doesn't .There are certain foods that do help with erections in men and some foods that do create lust in both sexes.

Take for example Oysters, good old oysters have been the cliche of all aphrodisiac foods for the ages. High in the mineral zinc which is a necessary requirement in the production of the male hormone testosterone and sperm. Oysters are also one of the most nutritional balanced foods containing proteins, lipid's, and carbohydrates. With their highest concentration of zinc, which is more than any other food,allowing 33mgs of zinc per serving its no wonder that just by eating several oyster's a day our libido begins to rise,and note that every time a man ejaculates he loses 2.5 mg of zinc and predisposes himself to prostate problems.

Sexual response does begin in the mind, and we have all said at one time or another that "I'm just not in the mood". The mind does play a dominate role in sexuallity. The center of the brain which issues commands has to be activated.

Hidden in the recesses of our hypothalamus and limbic system are intricate hormone receptors that bind with and are turned on by estrogen, progesterone, male hormones, prolactin, endorphins and possibly pheromones.
These and our brain cells don't get their information just from hormones but also from chemicals called neurotransmitters, dopamine, serotonin, and acetylcholine.We have

been told that the brain is our biggest sexual organ; hence its inclusion in this section. In normal circumstances sexual response requires messages from both the brain and the stimulated genitals. The brain's signals can be brought about by sight, smell, sound, and fantasy. These are processed in deep, primitive areas called the orgasm center.

Arousal may be even more brain-based than orgasm. Women, like men, have wet dreams: proof of a physical response prompted by our deep, or REM, sleep. But this is not common, and it would appear that for most of us, the threshold for stimulation of the brain is so high that it is difficult to achieve sexual fulfillment on brainpower alone.

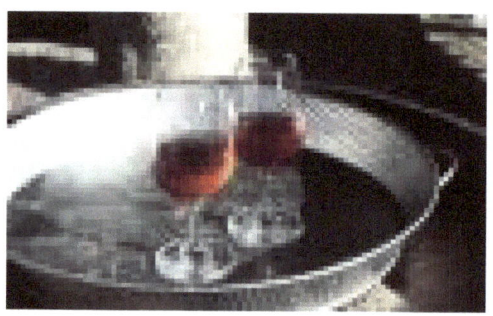

Sexual Frequency Chart
Intercourse Through The Ages Show That:

Percent of population having had first intercourse, by age:

Males	Females
25% by age 15	26% by age 15
37% by age 16	40% by age 16
46% by age 17	49% by age 17
62% by age 18	70% by age 18
69% by age 19	77% by age 19
85% by age 20-21	81% by age 20-21
89% by age 22-24	92% by age 22-24

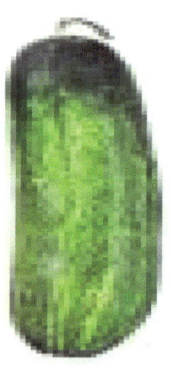

How Aphrodisiacs Affect Our Libido

There are more than 56% of women who are not functioning up to their sexual capacity. This incidence of decreased libido in the U.S. Ranges from adults in the percentage from 11 to 48%.Women are twice more likely than men to suffer from hypoactive sexual disorder,an aversion to steer away from any type sexual advance.

Sexuallity is an important way of life,but not in the sense of procriation,but a way of reinforcing sexual intimacy.When our sexuality is healthy, we often fail to notice how important it is. But when things aren't going well, bad sex may rule our relationship and indeed cause its demise. Sexual problems are a major reason for divorce, but the chicken-and-egg question is, "Which came first, a bad relationship, or bad sex?" Even in what the statisticians would call "normal" marriages, couples find that sex is disappointing or a downright failure 5 to 10 percent of the time.

Aphrodisiacs may influence our sense in certain deep areas of the brain that control our hormonal functions,and neurotransmitters. Now what better way to improve your sexual desire,health and techinque.Its the simplest recipe that creates all our sexual desires in a natural form that the body recognizes.

Their are also some doctors that use herbal and natural foods as treatments along with a clean healthy lifestyle to enhance one's sexual desires and treat impotence in men.

The simple sense of smell can also have an affect on men from women that can make some people stop and turn their heads. Phermones giving off by the body also affect our sexual senses.The sweat of a musculine man often wets the sexual apetite of a women,and in times of menstration during the menstrual cycle often does the same to men.

But according to science,it's all in the mind.If you think that something is an aphrodisiac,you then start behaving like its an aphrodisiac.I on the other hand tend to disagree with that statement,as I myself have tried and experienced the effects of certain aphrodisiac's only to discover the real truth,they do work !

However science doesn't know everything,so lets go and assume that aphrodisiacs work as per myth and legends say,but keep in mind that our brain is the biggest sexual organ.If you notice that some foods and herb's resemble certain sexual organs, bananas, cucumbers, ginseng, the mandrake, and some sea food, like oysters and mussels.

There are hundred's of acclaimed aphrodisiac's that science just labels them as folklore,but in truth many do have effects on certain regions of the brain that govern sexuallity.Many aphrodisiac's do contain nutritional factors that are highly rich in minerals,vitamin's,amino acids,hormone precursor's as you will later find out.Take the rhino horn for example and its phallic shape,which contains mostly phosphorus and calcium that when ingested may increase a sexual response in some individuals.

Most aphrodisiacs enhance aspects of the sensory experience such as ,smell,taste,sight,and hearing.Aphrodiciac's have a powerful affect on the mind as they are thought to trigger certain brain chemicals in the brain that stimulate certain organs.

An aphrodisiac keep in mind is a substance such as food,drug,herb,drink,or scent that can arouse or stimulate feelings of sexual desire.Named after the greek goddess of sexual love and beauty,Aphrodite.Bare in mind also that an aphrodisiac can be a stimulating full body massage or foot rub as well.Although it may seem like the last thing to stimulate the sexual senses,a foot massage can actually enhance sexual desire if done right.

Its the part of the brain that registers the sexual sensations a foot massage gives,is the same part of the brain that arouses sexual organs.Intensifying sexual arousal through the use of certain oils called "Aromatherapy" or "Essential Oils" like ylang ylang oil,or jasime oil can induce in some sexual sensations that induce sexual foreplay.There are many of these oil's that are quite effective in reducing stress which in turn releases tension thus freeing up your sexual desire.These concentrated oils work by stimulating the oflactory gland's sense of smell which is situated in the mucous membrane of the nasal cavity that sends signals to the hypothalamus.

About the size of a pearl,the hypothalamus directs a multitude of important functions in the body.The hypothalamus also influences various emotional responses linked to our sexual behavior.An integral part of the brain,the hypothalamus is linked with the pituitary gland in helping the human body maintain homeostasis,by regulating and producing various stress and sex hormones vital to our sexuallity.

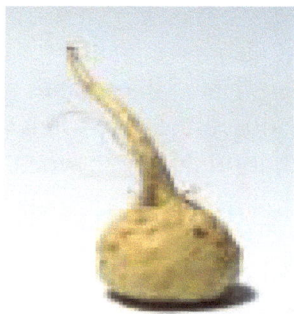

Herbal Aphrodisiac's That Work

Maca,. Lepidium meyenii – is Peruvian herb that grows in the high regions of the central andes.Maca was tradionally employed as an aphrodisiac and fertility ehancing capabilities.This acient nutritionally rich herb is used as a remedyand being dispensed by health care professionals as a safe and natural substitute for drugs.Doctor "Gloria Chacon" of Lima Peru,isolated four alkoloids from the root of maca and carried out animal studies with male and female rats showed multiple egg foliculle maturation's in the female rats,and in the male rats there were significantly higher sperm counts.Through the experiments she concluded that the alkoloids were acting on the hypothalamic-pituitary axis.Which explains why both male and female rats were affected.This also explains why the affects on humans are not limited to
the ovaries and testicles,but also on the stress glands of the adrenal glands giving one a feeling of high energy and vitality.

Today maca has been used for menopause,ferility,infertility,male menopause,
low libido and for increased sexual functions.Maca regulates the secretions of the internal organs,such as the pituitary,adrenals,thyroid,and the pancreas.Make sure you are buying the highest available extract possible,and maca comes in raw powder, and

capsules.

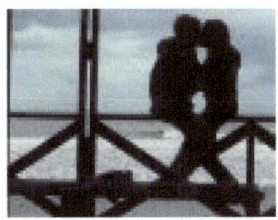

Tongkat Ali (eurycoma lonifolia) dubbed as the asian "viagra" in may 1999 in the New Sunday Times.It has been used by men in malaysia for its strong libido enhancing affect,sexual performance,and erectile dysfunction in men.
Also called "Man's Walking Stick" in malaysia,tongkat ali is a very interesting herb in that it does have drug like qualities in its fast affects.Tongkat Ali was traditionally used in malaysia for erectile dysfunction
and sexual potency,but its also beneficial in many other healthy ways as well,such as a popular remedy for malaria.

However,as for its use's today,the main usage of tongkat ali is focused for enhancing sexual drive in men and women.Tongkat is rapidly becoming world famous for its aphrodisiac qualities,but in america tongkat ali is somewhat new following the breakthrough of "viagra".
Tongkat ali works its effects by stimulating testosterone by freeing up the available free testosterone circulating in the blood stream.Most importantly,this extract has increased the formation of testosterone levels four fold in men,and increasing testosterone is the main objective from a sexual point of view.Women also produce testosterone,about 5% to 10% of what a man produces,but in women this vital hormone fans the flame of desire and increases the sensitivity in their erogenous zones,especially in their nipples and clitoris.Their sensitivity to the touch is sexually heightened.

By consuming tongkat ali,you can boost your testosterone levels back down to when you were young increasing your youthful levels and energy.With Tongkat ali you will maintain harder and stronger erections,your semen volume will increase,and you will attain stronger orgasm's.This herb comes highly recommended,cause I have witnessed the sexual affects for myself and its always the first one on my list of herbal supplements that I take personally for its testosterone boosting affect.It is so affective that even the bodybuilding crowd is using it to build their physique.Make sure the tongkat ali you purchase is of the sumatran brand and the extract is 200:1 but no less than 100:1 potency.When cosuming tongkat ali,it is recommended to cycle the herb for 4 weeks on and 2 weeks off at a time for its maximum benefit.

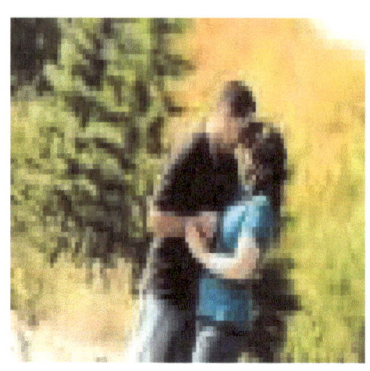

Tongkat Ali can be used by both men and women.

Horny Goat Weed (known as epimedium or ying yan huo) Behind the funny name of this remarkable herb stands a time tested aphrodisiac that has been used and prized by acient chinese text's.This herb increases libido in both men and women,and improves erectile dysfunction in men quite effectively.Today horny goat weed is gaining popularity around the world for its dramatic effect on libido and erections in men.This herb has long been employed to restore the sexual fire,boost erections,allay fatigue,and also as a nitric oxide stimulator in blood vasodilation.This plant got its name long ago when a goat herder noticed incessant sexual behavior in his goats after they were eating this one particular plant,and the goats promiscuous behavior became much worse and noticeable.

Horny goat weed works similar to the way the prescription drugs cialis and viagra work,studies indicate that horny goat weed works by increasing nitric oxide levels,which relaxes the smooth muscle tissues and lets more blood flow to the penis or clitoris.It also inhibits the PDE-5 enzyme,making it a PDE-5 class inhibitor like viagra and cialis.Icariin is the main active ingredient in horny goat weed.Most of the horny goat weed sold today is of a lower quality,say 10 to 20% standardization that generally takes time to take affect.But you can find higher extracts that are standardized to about 50% to 60% extractions on line on the internet..These are the ultimate strengths to look for,the higher the percentage of extract the quicker and faster the effects will be.Generally with these stronger types of extracts you will notice the affects to be similar to the sex drugs viagra and cialis,it works that fast ! Horny goat weed gives you back your sexual strength and vitality that you once had when you were young.

This is also a great herb to combine with tongkat ali for an even more potent mixture and effect that i'm sure you will be pleased with. ***Horny goat weed can be used by both men and women.***

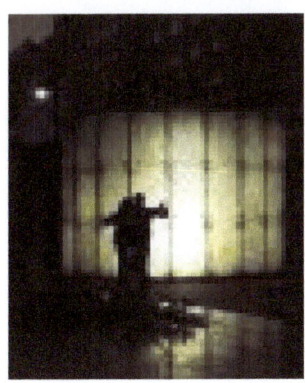

Clavo Hausca (tynanthus panurensis) is a highly regarded aphrodisiac for both sexes but especially
for women.It is widely sold and used for this purpose in Peru.The indian tribes of the amazon highly regard this plant for its remedy in male impotence and an effective aphrodisiac for women.Some women report that they become too sexually aggressive while on clavo when taking it on a daily basis.It is also reported to effective especially for pre-menopausal women,but not that quite effective for libido loss after menopause.As of the exact nature of how clavo works its magical aphrodisiac qualities on how it affects the brain is clearly not quite understood yet,more studies need to be had,but regardless its relatively a safe herb and no major side effects have been documented.
Clavo hausca is world renowned everywhere except but here in the US for its powerful aphrodisiac ,often being referred to as a "Women's Viagra".Although used by both men and women,it was used by the amazonian indians for weak erections in which they regarded it as highly effective.Though now its mostly used by women,because the effects are markedly stronger in women.Clavo does heightened the sexual response in women as there were a few studies done on this.It also induces strong vivid dreams of a sexual nature and has produced wet dreams in some women who were taking it on a daily basis.Preliminary phytochemical analysis done by brazilian scientists show an alkoloid they named "tinantina" as well as tanic acids,eugenol,and other essential oils.

Clavo can be taken in capsule,tincture,or as a decoction.There are extracts of a higher quality 10;1 ratio ,which should always be sought after.

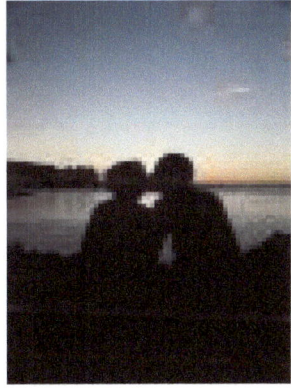

Butea Superba (Red Kwao Krua) this herb has been traditionally used to enhance erection quality.This heb is native to Thialand that has a characteristic of a crawling vine that wraps itself around large trees.The roots and stem of the plant have been used for strength and power centuries,and has been revered for its health producing abilities.Butea has also been used for medical research ,supplements,and for beauty treatment.the roots of the plant have been found to contain flavanoids,sterol compounds,and aldosterone which is a natural hormone thought to be an aphrodisiac.

Butea has a moleculor structure that makes it a natural PDE-5 inhibitor,thus making it a perfect natural male enhancer.research has it established that butea does facilitate a strong vasodilation effect with no side effects.This benefits males in multiple ways – supports blood flow to the male genitalia,promotes strong vasodialation affect via nitric oxide release,and ehances sexual sensitivity and performance.Enzymatic tests reveal it to be a potent inhibitor of c-AMP phosphodiesterase which reacts diretly on the corpus cavernosum in the penis enhancing blood flow to that area creating a more frequent ,longer lasting,stronger male sexual arousal peroid.Human trials do show it to be an effective erectile remedy for impotence.

One other study also showed it to have cholinergic activity,increasing acetylcholine levels in the body.Acetylcholine has also been noted to be involved in male erectile function and memory as well.Look for the highest standardized extract as possible when taken butea superba.

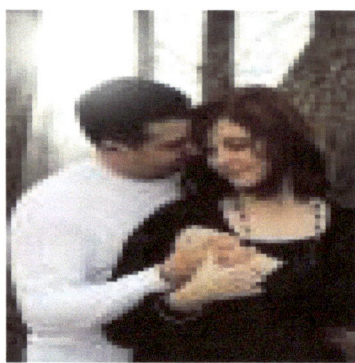

Xanthoparmelia Scabrosa – is an aphrodisiac useful in the treatment of male erectile dysfunction,that has found its way in many commercial aphrodisiac formula's sold in the market today.Its main function is that it induces smooth
muscle relaxation allowing for maximum arterial dilation of blood flow to the male gentitalia.
The chinese have known for decades that xanthoparmelia contains substances that greatly inhibit the production of the enzyme phosphodiesterase-V PDE-5
allowing for sustained erections.Xanthoparmelia supports erectile function ,and due to the fact that it greatly increases blood flow its alse used in bodybuilding in those seeking the "pump" during exercise.It works the body in a simular way that horny goat weed does but more effectively.This is another herb thats proven it's effectiveness when it comes to aphrodisiacs that work.The active extract one needs to follow is piperizine,make sure its standardized to 35% or higher if planning on using.

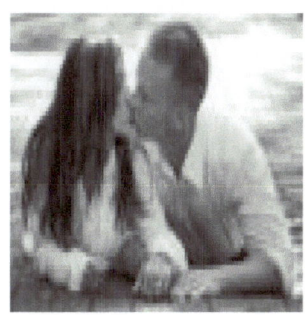

Cnidium Monnieri – a popular remedy in asian medicine for centuries,being first described 2,000 years ago.It naturally releases nitric oxide levels,increasing blood flow to the penis and clitoris.It is also useful for increasing the "pump" feeling during exercise.As a natural libido enhancer,cnidium has also been used in many of the popular libido enhancer's commly sold today,often combined with xanthoparmelia and horny goat weed which makes for a potent synergistic effect to enhance sexual desire and performance.The main active ingredient of cnidium is osthole,this herb also acts similar in affect to the current sex drugs levitra,viagra,and cialis.
Look for the highest extract available a 50:1 or higher if possible for the best sexual affects.Cnidium can be used by both men and women.

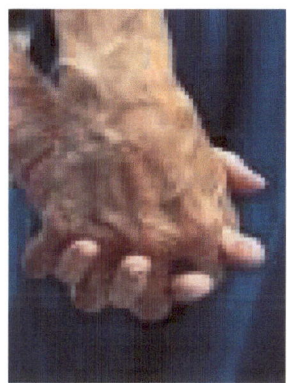

Kacip Fatimah – this herb is the female version of togkat ali.Despite its long history of traditional use,the active componets and mode of action have not been well studied although there is some preliminary research that has been published.Known as one of the premier herbal aphrodisiac in the world for women,kacip fatimah does have some beneficial effects that do benefit women after giving child birth.It supposedly restores the elasticity of the women's vagina after delivering a baby,inwhich I must attest that I have used this particular herb on my own wife and did defitnetly notice a difference in the tightness when having sexual intercourse.I'm sure after men read this they will go out and purchase as much kacip fatimah as they possibly can!

The way that kacip works its aphrodisiac affects is by making more free available testosterone,and in women they don't need much testosterone for them to get sexually aroused.This is one more herb that bare's researching as it has interesting qualities.I would look for the highest available extract and on line would be the proper place to look for.This herb has more of a specific affect on women than on men so I wouldn't bother using it for men.

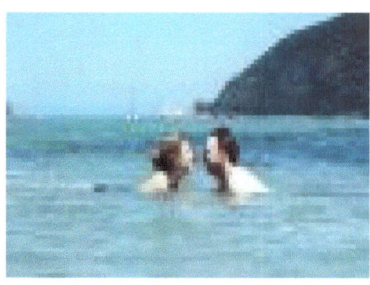

Dark Baker's Chocolate – I bet you never thought of this one,but pure chocolate has always been a common aphrodisiac that most people never thought of.Chocolate in most parts of the world has always been associated with romance and not without good reason.Originally it was viewd by the aztec's as an aphrodisiac who thoght that it would invigorate men and make women less inhibited.So when it was introduced in Europe,it was only natural that chocolate became the ideal gift to receive from a loved one or an admirer.

You may ask,what does this have to do with oysters,almonds,walnuts,and viagra ? Well,made from cocoa beans found in pods growing from the trunk to the lower branches of the Cacoa Tree.The Mayan civilation worshipped the tree for they believed it was from divine origin,thus its latin name Theobrom Cacao,meaning food of the god's. Cacao is a mayan word for god food.Chocolate is a very complex food that scientists have uncovered its secrets that when consumed it has a strange effect on humans.Chocolate contains two substances called Phenylthylamin and Seratonin, which have been noted for its mood lifting affect.Both of thes substances occur naturally in the brain when we are happy and also when we are experiencing feelings of love and passion.When eating chocolate,it gives an instant energy boost,increases stamina,and it is no wonder why its affects have given it a reputation as an aphrodisiac.Look for the more expensive chocolate thats sold today,it will have a higher percentage of cacao.The higher the better and quicker affects you will be assured of.There is nothing wrong with having a little pure chocolate with a glass of wine to set the tone for a romantic sexual encounter.

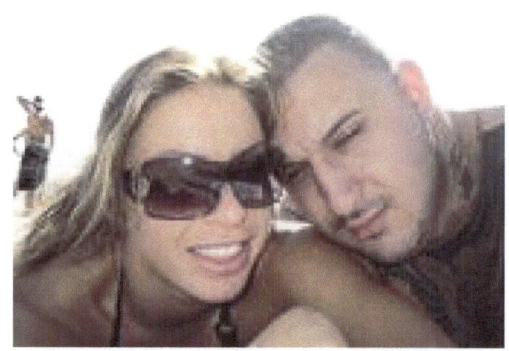

Yohimbe Bark **(corynanthe yohimbe)**– classified as the world's famous aphrodisiac .Yohimbe is an herb that has an affect on the human bodyas an aphrodisiac.A traditional African medicine thats been used as a treatment for leprosy,fevers,angina,and as a sexual treatment for sexual dysfunction.In europe it has been also used for more than 75 years as an accepted treatment for male erectile dysfunction.The bark of the yohimbe tree contains 6% of its active ingediate,yohimbine.It is the yohimbine that is used as the active componet in allopathic medications that are based on this herb's effectiveness.

It works by stimulating blood flow by dialating blood vessels,its this increase in blood flow to the penis that brings about the erections in men.Another manner relating to the effectiveness of this herb is that it increases the body's production of norepinphrine which is essential in the formation of of erections.In diabetic men,studies also show that this herb can restore the potency that they were suffering from impotence due to mainly of their disease.

Yohimbe when taken has a stimulating affect on sensory nerve endings that leads to a sexual sensation never before experienced.This I have noted for myself in experimenting with this classic herb,which at times to me was a bit overwhelming,but in most individuals trying it was a welcomed experience.
Just like anything else,some herbal aphrodisiacs will have different affects on different people.

Most of the yohimbe sold in health food stores today come in tablet,or capsule form with a standardized extraction of 6% or 8% strength.But it always pays to becareful as the strength of yohimbe can vary greatly,and may not always have the proper strength of the extract.Prescription yohimbe is another matter and that comes in a standard dose of 5.4 mgs.A typical dosage for erectile dysfunction would be 5.4 mgs three times aday.Anyone planning on taking yohimbe wether in a natural standardized dose or prescription should be aware of its side effects,like anxiety,nervousness,elevated blood pressure and allergic reaction.

Any individual should also be aware of not combining yohimbe with certain foods that contain tyramine,and that includes red wine,cheese,and liver.It should not also be used by anyone that has heart disease,kidney disorder,and liver disorder.So do your research just to be safe.For some individuals its a god send and highly favored,and for others not so.

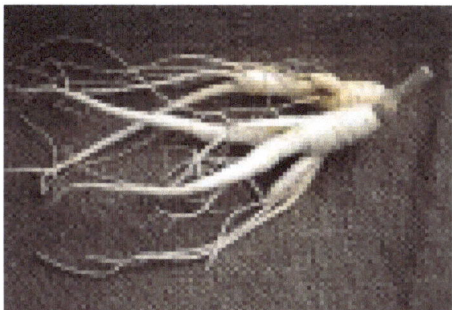

Korean Ginseng - (Panax quinquefolium) This very popular herbal has stood the test of time and just had to be included out of respect for its many beneficial health related properties,and its aphrodisiac affects as well.In animal studies,the purported effects of ginseng were substantiated when a biological basis for the claim of aphrodisiac was established.Ginsenosides were found to be directly involved in inducing a vasodilation and relaxtion effect on the penile corpus cavernosum.By dilating the blood vessels and relaxing the corpus cavernosum ,ginseng thus promotes erctions in men.A human experiment was done in an asian medical center ,60% of the men with erectile dysfunction reported that ginseng improved their erectile response.

Researchers also noted that ginseng also increased penile tip firmness during erectile response.Korean ginseng also has an indirect affect on nitric oxide levels,which is another explanation for its effectiveness in male impotence.

Ginseng primarily was used to restore homeostasis to the body which helps to explain its wide and beneficial effect in correcting many health related issues. Ginseng is a wide spread herbal machine thats has been used by the chinese for ages as a major componet for many chinese prescriptions in asian medicine.Look for the highest standardized extract when purchasing korean ginseng.This is one herb that I have used quite a many times when feeling run down and fatigued.

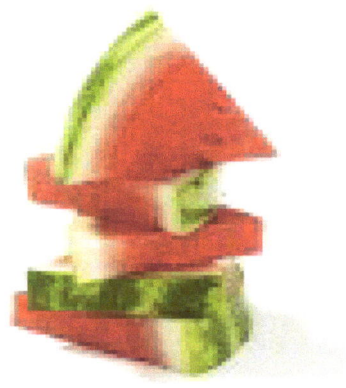

Aphrodisiac Foods That Stimulate Sexual Desire

Aphrodisiac foods go back as far as the romans and greeks to increase sexual power.During those peroids the people were concerned with fertility and sexual performance more so than passion itself,so a great amount of time was spent on determining what foods would help with these two concerns.So the realm of aphrodisiac foods got started and even today the most talked about legal aphrodisiacs come in edible form.As in acient belief systems as well as today,they saying still goes -you are what you eat,still holds true.

The aphrodisiac foods that are thought to be the most effective were usually chosen for their symbolic shapes associated with sex and sexuallity. While certainly not the most potent they are the easiest to access and in the right combination of aphrodisiac foods can help to jump start a very sensual evening.

The human libido is controlled by hormones,with testosterone being the key hormone and infuenced by certain key neurotransmitters,dopamine and serotonin.

If the balance is thrown off things may not function as well as they should.Testosterone production is dependent on zinc and B-vitamins,which are abundant in many foods.But as nutritional deficiencies decrease with age and lifestyle it needs these nutritional nutrients to replenish what has been lost. But there is some sound basic science about these various claimed foods that do increase libido,boost arousal,and put men and women in the mood.

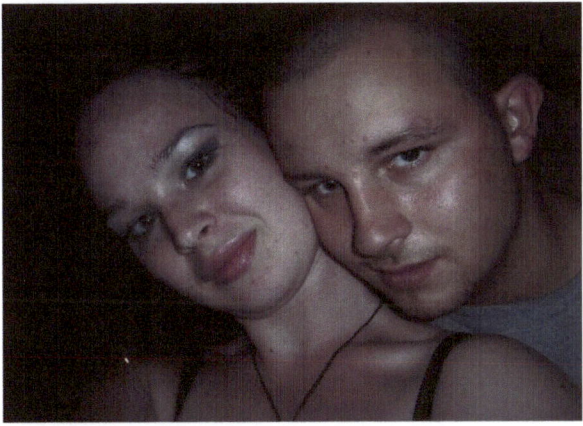

Watermelon – A study suggested that watermelon may have viagra like effects on the body.But the findings don't exactly mean that eating watermelon could boost libido or treat erectile dysfunction.Watermelon does contain large amounts of the amino acid "Citrulline",which is known to have favorable effects on the cardiovascular system and the immune system.Citrulline can relax blood vessels and improve blood flow in much the same way as the drug viagra does.

The researchers at Texas A & M's Fruit and Vegetable Improvement Center in College Station have made a wonderful discovery that may help cure erectile dysfunction and increase libido,that watermelon may be the new "viagra" on the block.As stated by Dr.Bhimi Patil at Teaxs A&M's research Center "The more we study watermelons,the more we realize what a amazing fruit it is in providing natural enhancers to the human body " and the list of benefits grows and grows.

Citrulline gets transformed into the amino acid Arginine after combining with certain enzymes within the body after waterm is consumed,and we know that arginine is a precursor to nitric oxide which helps dilate the blood vessels therefore boosting blood circulation.This has the same basic effect as viagra does in treating erectile dysfunction and mat even help prevent it.So give this tasty delicious fruit a try and see for your self.

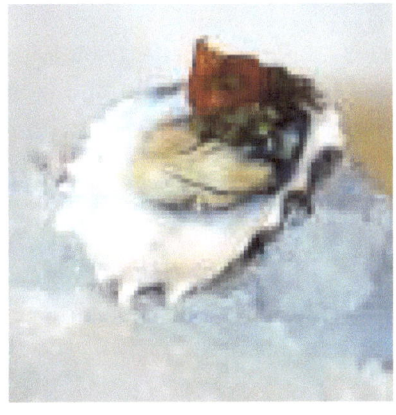

Oysters – Since acient times many people have considered oysters to a potent aphrodisiac food.It's reputation has arisen from the fact of its resemblance to the female gentitalia.However oysters do have a very high zinc content which is essential in the production of testosterone and in the maintenance of healthy sperm. But raw oysters are also high in the amino acid "D-aspartic acid" which increased testosterone levels in male rats in one study which could in theory increase libido.Also some oysters could change their sex from male to female and back,given rise to claim that the oyster lets one experience the masculine and feminine side of love.

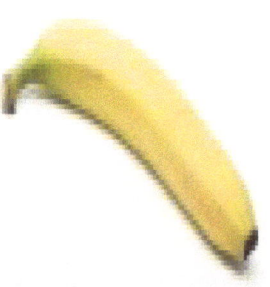

Banana's – This is a great energy given food source that contains the enzyme bromelain which is believed to improve the male libido.The phallic shape of the banana is partially responsible for the banana being a popular aphrodisiac.
Banana's however,are high in potassium and B-vitamins,especially B2,riboflavin which is also important in the production of testosterone.

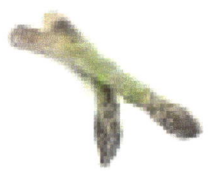

Asparagus – Known for its suggested shape,asparagus is high in the b-vitamin folate that aids in the production of histamine.Histamine is important
for a healthy sex drive in men and women.Also rich in vitamin E,which is essential for hormone-building,and it has been suggested by the Vegetarian Society that eating asparagus for 3 days will have a powerful affect to the human body.Asparagus also contains D-aspartic acid,healthy levels of potassium,magnesium,and phosphorus all which are healthy for high energy levels.In china, asparagus is considered a favorite sex food used for balancing weak kidney function.In the 17th century,an english herbalist "Nicholas Culpepper" wrote that asparagus "Stirs up the Lust in Men & Women"

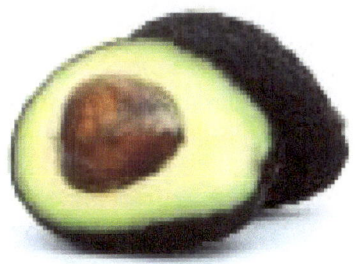

Avocado's – Just by looking at this fruit you can tell why the aztec's called the avocado "ahuacuati" or testicle tree. Which they thought that the fruit hanging from the tree resembled a pair of testicles.On the other side avocado's are rich in folic acid,B6,and potassium.Also loaded with essential fatty acid's which are necessary in the production of sex hormones,avocado may be a natural alterative to viagra.

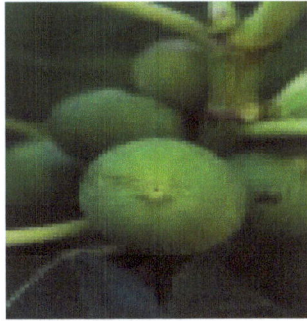

Fig's – this sexy fruit has long been thought as an arousing stimulant and opening it up is thought to emulate the female sex organs.Considered one of the oldest fruits in history regarded highly by cleopatra,and the acient greeks held them very sacred and associated them with love.Being high in amino acids which are critical in boosting libido and increasing your stamina.This tasty fruit is also rich in vitamins A,B,and minerals like phosphorus,iron,calcium,and manganese.

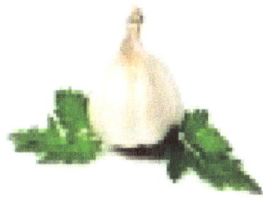

Garlic – not so well liked by some people because of its order,garlic offers a powerful kick to increase blood circulation,boost testosterone production,ward off illness,lower cholesterol and stimulates the immune system.The main ingredient in garlic,allicin a compound that can improve blood flow to the sexual organs that can improve erections in men.A study performed at St.ThomasHospital in the United Kingdom proved that by eating four cloves of garlic a day helped cholesterol levels and made room in the arteries for improved blood flow to the penis resulting in more erections.Garlic bad for the breath,but may be the equivalent to a natural viagra for men.

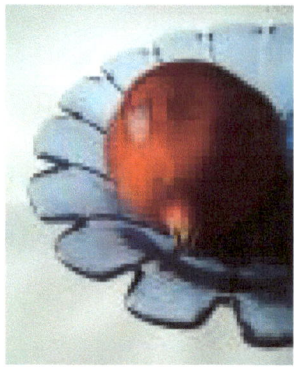

Pomegranate – This fruit bares some close paying attention too because of its powerful affect on blood circulation and other healthy benefits that is beginning to make the headlines as of late.It was noted that men and women who drank a glass of the fruits juice for a fortnight experienced a surge in testosterone,which increases sexual desire in both men and women.Lately claimed a super food,pomegranate would become to be known a natural aphrodisiac that works!

Previous research on pomegranate has determined it to be full of powerfull anti-oxidants which can help ward off disease and illness, and help boost blood circulation.The Edinburgh research measured blood testosterone levels in men and women which increased by 16% and 30% among the subjects tested.

New research revealed in a study of 53 male subjects with libido problems. After a month about 53% of the subjects said that their sexual performance increased after consuming pomegranate juice. It was also pointed out that pomegranate may help improve prostate cancer as well .This healthy juice with so many beneficial healthy effects would be on my kitchen table or refrigerator everyday of the week. Its tasty, healthy and serves as one of my favorite super foods and aphrodisiac's.

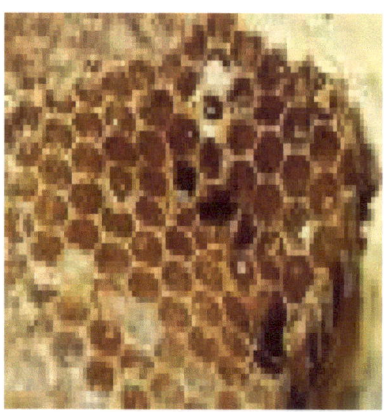

Natural Unfiltered Honey – A classic nutritional punch that is loaded with live natural enzymes, vitamins, minerals, and amino acids. Honey has been included in many aphrodisiac formula's in the recipe's that boost sexual desire and performance. One effective recipe taken before bedtime to stir the lust is a glass of honey together with a handful of almonds and pine tree nuts with a little bit of ground ginger was to be taken for three consecutive nights. Honey which contains bee pollen that may account for its sexual stimulating affect has been used through out the ages in so many cultures. It was also once said that if you put a women who's struggling to conceive on bee pollen,you can pretty much guarantee a result within two to three months. The belief is that the bee pollen increases the biological value of the egg, restoring and rejuvenating natural hormonal substances within the body.

A beverage of honey and water was also once a natural aphrodisiac taken before any sexual encounter.

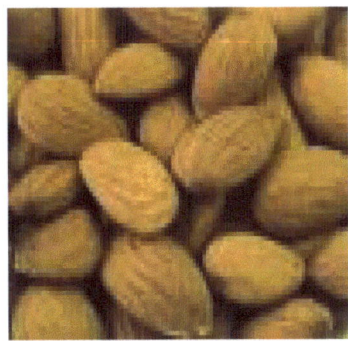

Almonds- Throughout the ages almonds have been a symbol of fertility one of the oldest known aphrodisiacs and fertility symbols. With its high value of the amino acid L-Arginine,which helps relax blood vessels and improve circulation,also rich in vitamin E and essential fats, almonds have always been linked to a good healthy sex life. Raw or roasted almonds are the healthy option here. In India,they use the kernel of the almond in healing premature ejaculation. The aroma of almonds was also thought to stimulate the passion in women,and the scent of almonds is one of the most all time favorites in the pursuit of love and seduction. Just eating a handful of raw almonds before bedtime can bring about an erection in men. We know also have almond butter and almond milk which now are two healthy alternative foods that we can combine to spruce up a romantic sexual encounter in   the recipe of love.

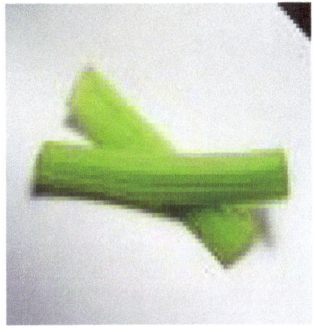

Celery – While celery may not be an aphrodisiac food that comes to mind when it pertains to thinking about sex,It can be a fantastic food source for sexual stimulation. This is because it contains "Androsterone" ,an orderless hormone that is released by a man's perspiration that is often said "turns women on".Androsterone is in fact a product of the metabolism of the male hormone testosterone and probably an important link in the chain of the breakdown of the male androgen hormones into chemicals like andro-phermones, androstenone, and androstenlone.

Celery is in fact a high fiber low calorie food,83% water with essential minerals like sodium, calcium, magnesium, zinc, iron, phosphorus, and as well as vitamins A, B, and C. It makes for a healthy snack besides for improving one's sex life.

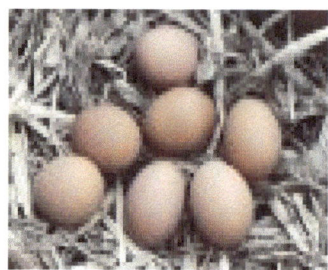

Eggs – Not one of the most sensual foods thought of as an aphrodisiac, eggs are high in nutritional value and are one of the most biological foods high in B5,B6, lecithin, acteylcholine, and amino acids. Which help the body balance vital hormones and stress that are so crucial in maintaining a healthy sex drive. Eggs have also been a symbol of fertility and strength throughout the ages. Some people will eat raw eggs just prior to a sexual encounter to increase their sexual libido and performance. All bird and chicken eggs contain a good amount of vitamins B5,and B6.A good healthy snack before love making would be some caviar,and a small glass of champagne with some ha
Rd boiled eggs.

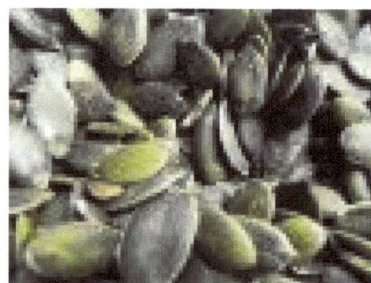

Seeds & Nuts – just like oysters, pumpkin seeds, and pine nuts are a rich source of zinc, which help the body produce testosterone and sperm. Nuts are a good source of essential fatty acids which help to prevent plaque accumulation in the arteries and improve blood flow throughout the body, especially to the genital region. Further more nuts and seeds are power house foods that are full in protein and healthy fats which can give you a boost in the bedroom.

Conclusion

Author's Personal Favorite Top Five Aphrodisiac's

Herbal Aphrodisiac's
(1)   Tongkat Ali
(2)   Horny Goat Weed
(3)   Korean Ginseng
(4)   But Superb
(5)   Xanthoparmelia

Top Five Aphrodisiac Foods
(1)   Watermelon
(2)   Almond's
(3)   Egg's
(4)   Honey
(5)   Pomegranate

In closing I would like to add that modern science may say what they may, about aphrodisiacs. In truth its been said many of times that we are what we eat, and History would not lie in revealing the truth's to many of these natural sources of herbal and food aphrodisiac's that have been used throughout history and stood the test of time. I myself have witnessed the effects of these natural aphrodisiac's only to be impressed by their delivery and satisfaction. I have done the research for you and have listed what I've thought to be   the aphrodisiac's that work and have the effect that they claim. So,you be the judge and enjoy the many wonderful affects of nature as it would be. Good health to all,and enjoy discovering the wonderful world of aphrodisiac's.

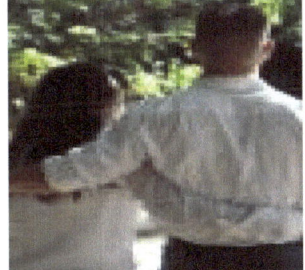

Of all nature's secrets the pursuit of natural aphrodisiac's that do work have been sought out by man looking for that special something to fan our flame's seeking the sexual bliss that nature can provide.

Based on herbs and natural foods, the aphrodisiac's listed in this book provide you with most select choice's that do work in enhancing sexual desire. This book informs you of they can help you nutritionally and sexually. It's goal is to help you also get the most out of your libido in choosing over 20 aphrodisiac's that can greatly enhance your sex life.

This book is also an excellent resource for those seeking to educate themselves in the history, effectiveness, and safety of natural aphrodisiac herb's and foods. With the prescription drugs that treat erectile dysfunction today it would nice to seek something more simpler, cheaper and natural that can have the same effect but in a natural sort of way.

With details of how natural substances can contain vitamins, minerals, essential fatty acids, and amino acids that have a reputedly profound and beneficial effect towards enhancing your libido. To all you lover's out there, there is a safe choice in stimulating your passions,"Aphrodisiac: Proven Sex Boosters For Men & Women That Do Work" is the book you need to read.